Come On Beautiful, Move!

Real Moves That Will Change The Course Of Your Life

Come On Beautiful, Move!

Real Moves That Will Change The Course Of Your Life

Nikki K. Conley, MPH

Copyright © 2017 by Nikki K. Conley

ISBN-13: 978-1548569051   1548569054

info@healthquestsolutions.org

www.healthquestsolutions.org

Book cover design by Maurice Ingram
Illustrations by Lauren Glover

Thank you, Christ, for your blessings and new mercies.

Contents

Afterwards by Tissilli Rogers

Chapter 1

Either you will or you won't (take care of yourself).

Let's start out by stating the obvious. We are on this earth for a very limited time. Pastor Dale Bronner once said, "We are born looking like our parents, but we die looking like our decisions." It is a fact that the decisions you make today will undoubtedly have an impact on what happens to you in the future. Or, it could be said that the decisions you made in your past are affecting you right now. Whichever way you chose to look at this, you must realize *you* are living with the results of your own decisions.

We come to this Earth to live and learn the lessons life has to offer. However, between the time we are born and die there is a lot of work to be done. This work may not be your calling, but we all have a job to do. You may be a mother, a teacher, an accountant, a doctor, a dancer, etc. Whatever your job or calling may be, you must be healthy to be effective.

For example, if you are an attorney, your clients expect you to be in beast mode when you represent them in a court of law. They need all of you. How can that happen if you are unable to adequately produce because of the unhealthy lifestyle choices you made? No one wants an attorney who is missing court or not prepared for cases because they are constantly struggling with an illness that could have been prevented with better lifestyle choices.

Some of these preventive illnesses include type II diabetes, heart disease and stroke. According to the U.S. Department of Health and Human Services Office of Minority Health, four out of five African American women are overweight or obese. Unfortunately, that means African American women struggle with their weight--and all the health problems that come with it-- more than other group of men or women in America. ("Obesity and African Americans," June 27, 2016). Given the many significant ways African American women have lead this county, this statistic is ironically tragic.

African American women have led the way for this great nation in many prolific ways. Astronaut Dr. Mae Jemison, entertainer Lena Horne and politician Shirley Chisholm are just few of the women whose leadership and legacy have profoundly affected and influenced this nation. However; even with the great minds, voices, barrier breakers and leaders this nation has produced, African American women lead the way in many unhealthy categories as well.

Before we go any further, let's get one thing straight. The purpose of this book is not to harp on the gloom and doom that affects so many in the African American community. Yes, I could write a whole dissertation on access to affordable health care, lack of healthy food options in some communities and the importance of eliminating the many health disparities and inequities that continue to plague our community. The focus could be on all the problems (and there are certainly a lot), but I'd much rather focus on the solutions that can bring about real change.

So the question must be asked, will you or won't you decide to take care of yourself? Will your life be filled with excuses or execution? Whichever option you chose--excuses or execution--both require a plan. You can plan to make excuses as to why you can't or don't have time to exercise. Some of the most common excuses—"I work a lot and I just can't fit exercise in." Or, "After I get off work, I have to get home, cook dinner and tend to my kids." Or my favorite, "I woke up too late" (and every day tends to be a late wake up day for these individuals).

Trust me, I get it. There is a lot on your plate as a wife, mother, career woman, and entrepreneur. However, at some point, you must stop and ask yourself, "Is this healthy for me?"

There are also real barriers that can prevent one from getting the proper physical activity they need. Some of these barriers include the financial costs (joining a gym or the YMCA), lack of motivation or a simple lack of knowledge. Some women may not see themselves as overweight or obese and may simply see themselves as "thick chicks." Moreover, some women may not have a babysitter or someone dependable to watch their children while they work out. All these barriers are real--particularly for single mothers who are shouldering all of the primary parenting responsibilities in their family.

Perhaps you are "The Quintessential Strong Black Woman." We all know how the story goes--I take care of everybody else and my concerns and interests come last, if at all. You *are* "Superwoman." You're constantly working to meet your family's needs and your boss expectations; still, your personal goals fail to meet your own standards of excellence.

Stop. It's time to change. Please, don't do this to yourself. In reality, if something happens to "Superwoman," her family has no idea how to function as they try to do all the things "Superwoman" use to do. But, they figure it out. Don't be mistaken. I know you are strong and your strength may be critical to those who rely on you. But at some point, you must put some *other* critical things first--your heart health, your sanity, your personal health and physical well-being. If you don't, the consequences can be detrimental.

To avoid those consequences, you must have a plan. Remember, it's either going to be excuses or execution. If you need help executing a plan to get on track and to stay on track, keep reading this book. Many solutions will be offered to help you live a long, healthy, positive and fun life. Life is short, neither the rest of today nor tomorrow is promised to us. So, if you are going to live, let's choose to live a great and healthy life today.

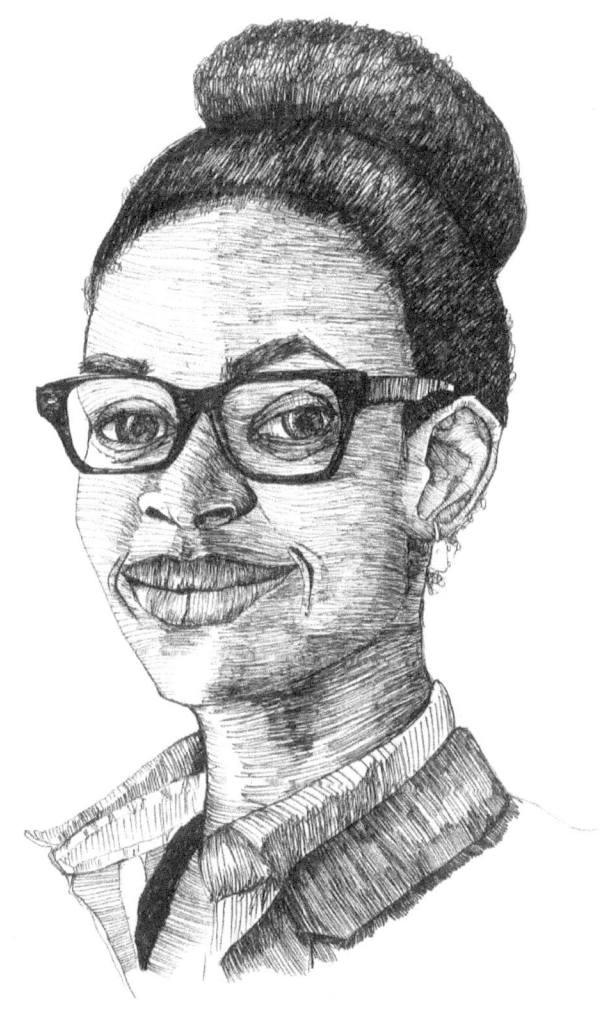

Chapter 2

Where's the little girl who use to play?

Tag, you're it! Let's race! How about a game of kickball? Do you remember saying those things as a little girl? Or even better-- actually playing those fun games with childhood friends? Do you remember going outside to play or maybe even having recess at school? Unfortunately, in this day and age, many children do not have recess at school. Some kids don't even bother going outside to play. But many of us did have recess and we enjoyed having time to run and play. To be clear, physical education class is something totally different from recess. This will be discussed in a later chapter.

Whatever happened to playtime and having good 'ol fashioned fun? I know we grow up, start working, get married, have children, then one day we realize we forgot how to play. We forgot how to take care of ourselves. We forgot how to nurture our own basic needs. The truth is, no matter how old we get, we still have a little girl who lives inside of us. That little girl longs to live a wonderful life and have a good time doing it. She wants to play!

From my experience working as a health and physical education teacher in elementary, middle, and high schools, by the time African American girls reach around seventh grade, many-- but, certainly not all of them-- want nothing to do with physical education or running around at recess. I have often asked myself, "What's up with this? Why won't my little African American sisters fully participate in class?" It upsets and saddens me because I know the extraordinary befits of exercise. But more importantly, I know what preventable sicknesses and diseases they put themselves at risk for if they don't incorporate fitness activities into their lives. For many young girls, there is no one at home modeling what it's like to be a part of a family that regularly participates in physical activity.

There are always exceptions. But when I ask my students if they walk or do any type of exercise with their parents, the majority say they do not. So again, the healthy behavior is not demonstrated at home. I am not placing the blame completely on parents. It's very plausible that their own parents did not model the behavior for them.

Here's the good news. As Black women, we can solve this problem. First, we need to get families to do something as simple as walking together after dinner and not just sitting in front of the television, tablet, cell phone, or any other device that distracts us from exercising. This is just one of many steps that can help reduce the rate of diseases and disorders that disproportionately affect our community.

Now, I know this may sound incredibly simple or even naïve. And I get it; unfortunately, some of our neighborhoods may not be the safest areas to go for a walk or a jog. But allow me to make a suggestion. Keep a pair of tennis shoes in your vehicle. When you take your children to their afterschool sports activities, grab your sneakers and walk around the perimeter of their practice field or court. I think you will agree, this is a much healthier option than just sitting there checking your email or updating your Facebook or Instagram page. It also eliminates the excuse that "I don't have time" because you have as much time as your son or daughter has on the practice field.

Another thing you can do on your own is use your cell phone, computer or tablet, to help you work out. If you can't hire a personal trainer, get on Youtube.com and find a workout routine.

There are literally thousands of exercise routines on Youtube.com that you can use to workout. Best of all--it's the cost of you paying your cell phone or internet bill.

There are high and low impact routines, dance workouts and many other kinds of exercise routines on the internet. However, just because someone has a YouTube channel does not mean they are reputable or knowledgeable. Make sure to check their background to determine if they have some type of certification or can demonstrate they have expertise in the area of fitness instruction they are providing. But before you take any action, consult a physician to ensure you are healthy enough to start an exercise program.

Back to the topic at hand, now that you're a fully grown woman, remember that little girl who use to love to run, play, jump rope and beat the boys in basketball? You know she's still in there, right? You take care of everything and everybody else, so why not take care of her? Why not help her push harder to prevent being overweight and obese, having a stroke, or developing hypertension and coronary heart disease? The choice is yours!

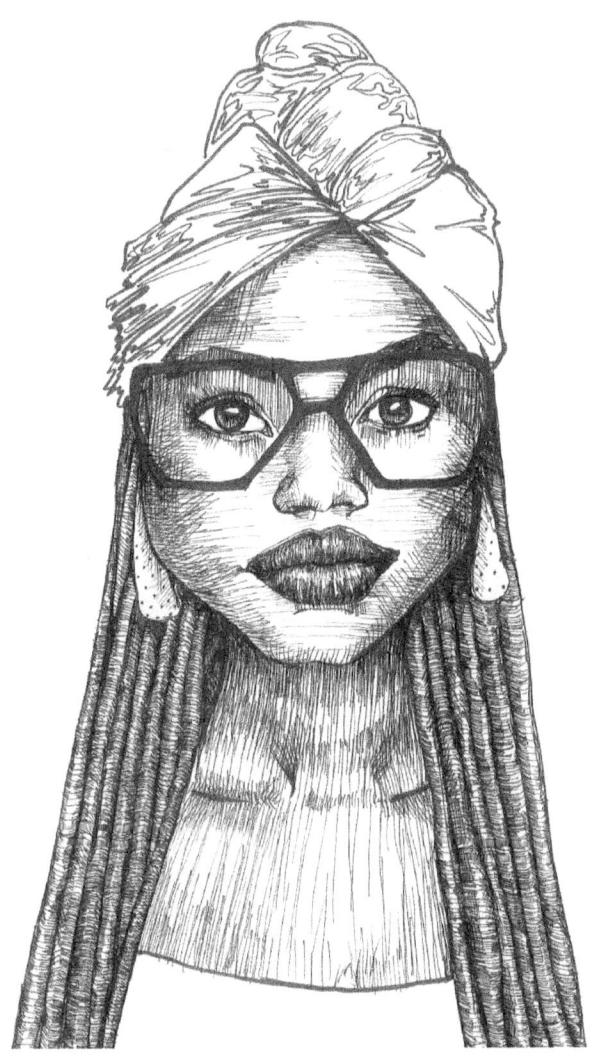

Chapter 3

Are you really your hair?

In 2005, India.Arie released a beautiful song-anthem called, "I Am Not My Hair." She sings about the journey she has taken with her hair. After what appears to be much self-reflection, she eventually comes to the realization that she is not her hair, she is so much more.

A Black woman and the connection to her hair can be complicated and difficult. But at the same time, it can be beautiful and intriguing. We love our hair, especially after we have just gotten it done. Even when we may be feeling down, after sitting in our hair stylist's seat and seeing the miracles he or she put together, we feel like a gorgeous beauty queen. A women's hair is her crowning glory. Unfortunately, for African American women it is also a major constraint.

According to a study done in 2013 by Hall, Francis, and Whitt-Glover, research suggests concerns related to maintenance of hairstyle (including styling time and financial cost to maintain hairstyle) were significant barriers to physical activity for many African American women. Some participants reported spending a good deal of time and money to maintain certain hairstyles, which can quickly become undone by sweating. Thus, these women may feel hesitant to participate in activities that involve physical exertion, given their desire to preserve their hairstyles for as long as possible (Pekmezi, D. Marcus, B. and Meneses, K., 2013). In other words, sistas don't want to sweat out the hairstyle they just spent hours of time and lots of money to get done. But this rationale can be detrimental to our health when you consider the significant economic burden of obesity and obesity-related diseases (Gathers, R. and Mahan, M., 2014).

If it were possible to run to the hairdresser after every workout, we might be inclined. However, for most of us this is simply not a realistic option. So what is a Black girl to do? Let's start with what many researchers have concluded. African American women who wear natural styles are more inclined to work out than those who wear their hair in chemically straightened or pressed out styles. Natural hair is defined as hair that has not been chemically altered by a perm or texturizer. I understand everybody is not going to rock an afro, twist out or any other natural style. No judgement. Wearing your hair in a natural style is simply an option that could be considered.

As another alternative, I highly recommend protective styles (as in weaves or braids). Just keep in mind, they can be positive and negative. If you have or can find a beautician who can braid or cornrow your hair without excessively tight pulling and causing tension on the scalp, then braids are a great alternative. But please be aware that if your stylist is pulling your hair too tightly, after wearing these styles for a number of years, traction alopecia can develop. This form of baldness happens over time after continued pulling on the hair and scalp. This pulling usually occurs around the temples or front hairline.

Another type of alopecia that has been linked to weaves, braids and tension or similar type styles is Central Centrifugal Cicatricial Alopecia also known as CCCA (Pallarito,K.,2011). CCCA hair loss starts to occur at the crown of the head. Treatment is available if identified in the very early stages. If you do notice any type of hair loss or hair thinning, seek immediate consultation from a dermatologist.

Unfortunately, these are some of the consequences that may occur if we are not careful about the protective styles we use for our hair. The key here is to find a trusted, well-trained and experienced stylist who specializes in quality hair care—not just hairstyling.

I know firsthand--the struggle is real for Black women and our hair. Our hair plays a major role in how we look and feel about ourselves. We pay a lot of money to keep our hair tight and looking right. However, there comes a time when we must look ourselves in the mirror and ask if we are truly happy with what we see in our reflection. If you're sick or on the verge of being diagnosed as a pre-type II diabetic, or type II diabetic with hypertension, overweight or obese and possible heart disease, what difference does it really make if your hair looks great? Again, these illnesses can be prevented. Please don't let your hair hold you back from living a full and healthy life.

For my sisters who perm or press their hair or wear blow outs, this is not an attack on you. According to the Hall, Francis and Whitt-Glover study, African American women with relaxed hair were more likely to avoid exercise because of their hair. Straightened hair should no longer stop you from working out and being healthy. There are products that some women with straight hair use and they find them to be helpful when working out. There are head wraps that can hold the hair in place and some of these wraps have moisture wicking technology and their purpose is to preserve the hair style while working out.

If your hair is long enough, pull it back in a ponytail, put the wrap on and go exercise. As a matter of fact, try something bold every now and then. On the day that you're going to get your hair done or the day before you get it done go swimming or exercise in a pool. Just for a day, try something different. Look at Olympic swimmer Simone Manuel. She won the 100 Free Style and became the first African American women ever to win an Olympic gold medal in swimming. Consider how great you could be if you just get your hair wet.

Please, let's not allow hair to continue to be a barrier for us not exercising on a consistent basis. It's just not worth it. What's the point in having gorgeous luxurious hair but you're sick in the doctor's office or hospital with preventable diseases? Or worse yet-- who has ever said, "Girl your hair is beautiful. I know you can't see it because of the damage that diabetes has caused to your eye sight, but trust me it's hot." Let me clear being sick is no fun.

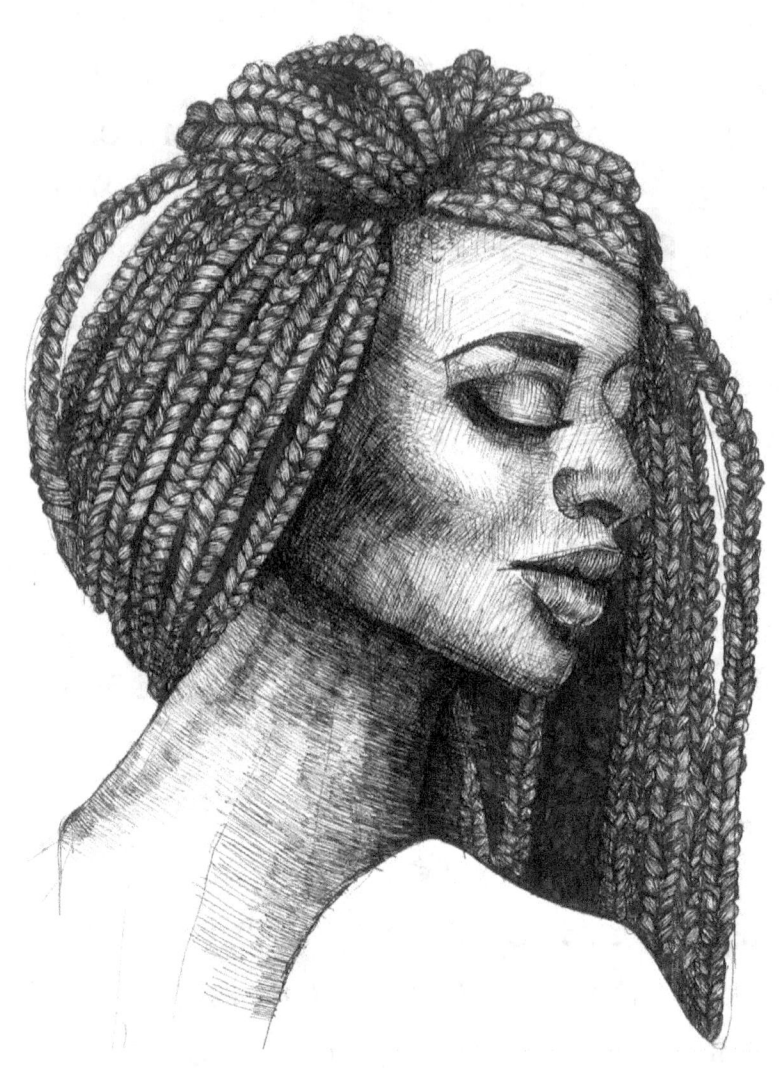

Chapter 4

Yo momma so fat!

"Yo momma so fat, she has to iron her pants in the driveway." "Yo momma so fat, she takes baths in the Atlantic Ocean." Growing up, we called this fun and entertaining discourse joaning. In other parts of the country, joaning is also known as playing the dozens, snaps, or woofing. One of the best way to get under someone's skin while joaning was to disrespect their mother and talk about how fat and ugly she supposedly was. No matter what may have been said during these verbal battles, a good "yo momma so fat" line was a sure way to get a great laugh.

But this is no joking matter. Our mothers, grandmothers, daughters, aunts, cousins and friends are in a crisis. Being fat, obese and overweight has physical, social, and emotional complications.

Mommies mean everything to the family unit—especially in the Black community. They work tirelessly to ensure their children and everyone else is taken care of and all their needs are met. For most of us, mothers are the ones who prepared the meals we ate. They bought the food that was in the refrigerator, freezer and pantry. This obesity problem is not just solely a lack of will power. There are some very powerful influences working against you.

Food is supposed to nourish your body. But as you may be aware, the food industry has changed over the years. There are quite a few documentaries and books that illustrate this. So yes, exercising is extremely important. But our food choices are equally—if not more important. We need to take a buyer's beware attitude before most food even reaches our mouth.

For example, did you know that some ice cream products can no longer be called "ice cream?" What a lot of people call "ice cream" is actually categorized by the U.S. Food and Drug Administration as "frozen dessert" depending on its contents. It gets complicated, but I will try to explain.

According to Title 21 of the FDA's Code of Federal Regulations, ice cream must contain no less than 10 percent milkfat. There are also specific guidelines for how much sugar and fat must be used to manufacture ice cream. Even the final weight of the product determines if it can truly be defined as ice cream. Frozen desserts do not have to meet these same guidelines.

When I was coming up, Breyers use to be known as the "all-natural" ice cream brand. My mother would always buy it when it went on sale because she said it tasted very similar to her grandmother's homemade ice cream. Currently, even Breyers sales some of its products as frozen desserts. Now, I don't know the science behind all the change that is taking place in the food industry, but I am pretty sure some of it boils down to cutting down production costs.

Let's take a look at another product I find absolutely ridiculous. It's has been marketed extremely well and people love it: Vitamin Water. When I first learned of this beverage, I was perplexed and wondered why would anyone buy a product called Vitamin Water. Why wouldn't you just drink water and take a vitamin? It's simple and would be a whole lot cheaper.

These two examples speak volumes as to how the food and beverage industry has done a great job in marketing products. Take a look at the numerous commercials on television and on line. You hardly ever see commercials telling you to go buy carrots or celery. You may occasionally see an advertisement for Washington Apples or some other fruit, but the marketing for healthy food pales in comparison to advertisements for fast food, soda, sugary cereal and potato chips.

A lot of this processed food is filled with salt, fat, sugar and a tremendous amount of artificial flavoring. I believe these foods can be addictive because sometimes you literally cannot eat just one.

Don't be fooled by the term "all natural." The FDA definition allows for parameters, but it seems the "all natural" label can be used very liberally. We also may never know what chemicals have been sprayed on our fresh fruits and vegetables. I would love to suggest you eat only organic products, but that can be expensive. Buying non-organic fruits and vegetables is fine, but please wash and soak them in apple cider vinegar, which works as a non-toxic cleanser. Pray over your food and let it nourish your body.

We can't live in fear, but we must be very intentional about the food and drinks we consume.

I say all of this, because I want you to get active and live a full life. But I also believe Americans have been bombarded and bamboozled by the food and beverage industry. For example, I asked my daughter the other day not to eat any more sweets she received in a goody bag. She responded by making a case that fruit snacks were not that bad because they were **fruit snacks** and questioned what could be better for a kid than fruit in a snack form.

It is quite baffling how we, as Americans, have gotten to this point. But for the sake our health, our bodies and our children, African American women must be the agents of change to reverse some of these disturbing health trends.

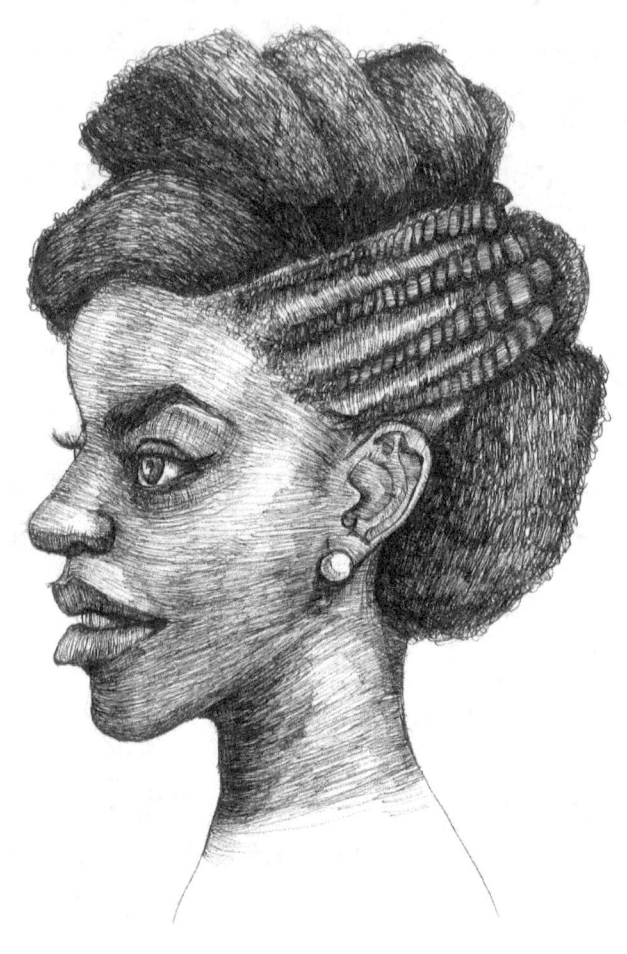

Chapter 5

Hold physical education teachers accountable.

The physical education (PE) teacher can a be very valuable resource. Even if you do not have children or your children have long finished grade school, physical education teachers can truly make a world of difference when they are held accountable. Unfortunately, the reputation of some physical education teachers leaves much to be desired. Let me elaborate a little bit more.

Regrettably, some physical education teachers just don't do their job. They roll the balls out and they don't teach the students a darn thing. They play every class period. Here's a scenario I've seen many times in my experience as a physical education teacher. The boys will be on the basketball court playing ball and the girls will be sitting in the bleachers talking, doing hair or reading a book. Absolutely no physical education is taking place at all. This is not what a physical education class should look like. It is actually quite disgusting.

One of the most important jobs of the physical education teacher is to teach fitness skills that can be used throughout life. It's like the math teacher who shows students how to add and subtract. These are skills a student will have for a lifetime. The physical education teacher should strive to do the same. Teach students lessons that will last a lifetime.

I have worked in several schools and I have seen some egregious acts of so called "teaching." I believe you should be the type of teacher who runs the type of classroom you would want your own child to attend. I can honestly say there were one or two individuals I have worked with whom I would not want in front of my children's class. It was not because these people were mean to the students or that they were bad people, they were just awful teachers. Terrible.

They had been teaching for many years and had become disgruntled. It was sad. They were no longer full of joy and they complained about everything. This is the most dangerous type of teacher because when someone gets to this point, there is not much teaching that will be taking place. Guess who suffers? That's right, your child.

Some might say, "It's just physical education class. Why are you taking it so seriously?" I take it very seriously because the physical education class can be a real tool to help kids reach their optimal health. The physical education teacher's classroom should be an asset to the educational environment. It should enhance student's development, not take away. I have seen many obese and overweight children during my time as a physical education teacher. My job was to teach the importance of health, wellness, nutrition as well as to get them to move and have fun doing it. A physical education teacher really does a disservice if they simply roll the balls out. This is just playtime and not a real physical education class.

One mistake that I have seen take place especially amongst male physical education teachers is they treat every student the same. This is fine when students are younger or in elementary school, but things change quite a bit for some girls when they reach middle and high school. They start to develop breast, waistlines and a back side. That's part of the reason why it can become extremely uncomfortable working out in front of hormone-enraged, horny, girl crazy preteen and teenaged boys. Some teachers simply are not sensitive to the needs of their students. These teachers will carry on with their lesson and won't even try to determine why a student is not participating or dressing out for class. They would just assume "let'em flunk."

Physical education teachers also should not make everything a competition. I have heard several young ladies- usually in middle school and high school- say to me, "I am not athletic and that's why I don't like P.E. class." In past classes, many of these young ladies were forced to compete and play against aggressive boys and it was not a positive experience for them. Instead of being a physical education teacher, many of these people are coaches who don't know when it's time to take the coaching hat off and teach a P.E. lesson.

For these reasons, I am a huge proponent of all girl physical education classes starting around seventh grade. Some school systems already offer this, but many do not. When girls don't have to worry about silly boys making crazy comments, and leaving them feeling insecure, they do better. Of course, parents play a major role in their children's well-being, but good physical education teachers can set children on a path of lifelong healthy behaviors as well.

If you need help coming up with exercises and you don't have the money to hire a personal trainer, put the physical education teacher to work at your child's school. The P.E. teacher can work for both you and your children. Ask him or her to help guide you and your child. They can do some of the things a hired personal trainer can do, like develop and write up a workout plan for you and your child.

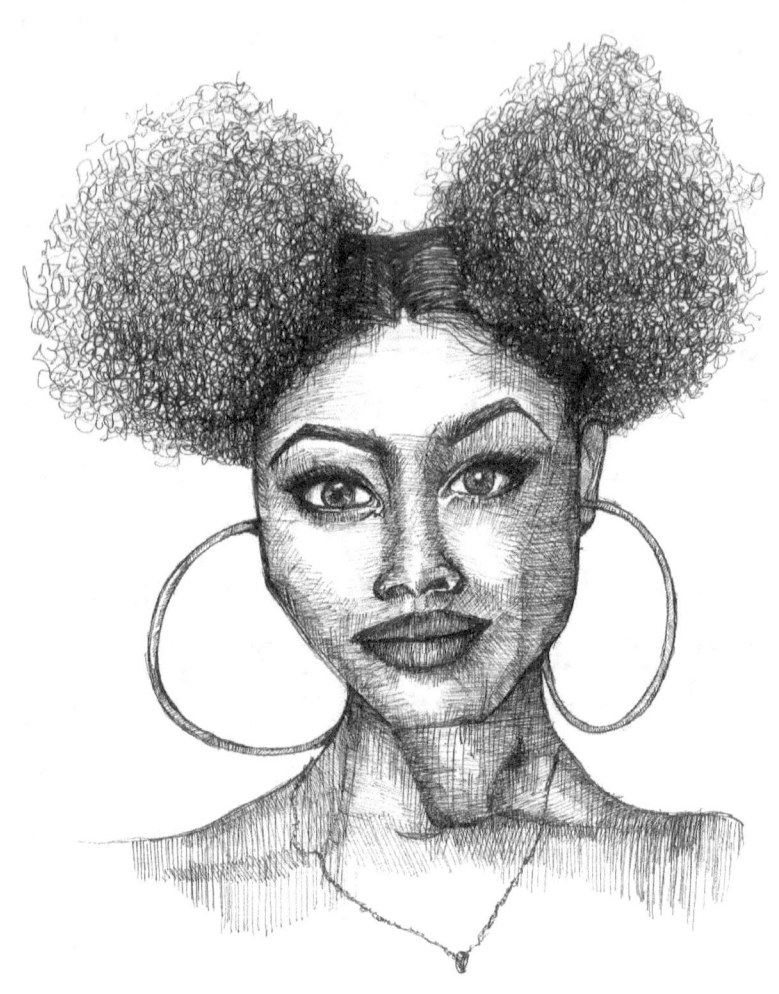

Chapter 6

Nothing's wrong with a thick chick.

A thick chick: not too fat and not too skinny. Thick and just right in all the right places. There is nothing wrong with being thick. As a matter fact, many brothers say they like a woman with some meat on her bones. For many African Americans, being too skinny is frowned upon and considered undesirable. Let's face it. There are plenty of celebrities who want what our mothers gave us naturally. Sir-Mix-A-Lot praised Black women about it in the early 1990's with his hit song, "Baby Got Back." Thick chicks—it's what's hot and poppin'.

But what happens when you are one burger away from no longer being just a thick chick? What comes after thick chick? Sorry to say this, but it's fat a chick with a host of health problems. There is quite a bit of research that shows African American women have different views of what is acceptable weight compared to our White counterparts. Simply stated, they may not see themselves as overweight or obese. They see themselves as just thick or even big boned.

Yes, it is true that people have different sized bones. Of course, we are not all the same height, we have different frames and different bone density, but that is not going to make a true difference in your weight. So, saying you are big boned is just talk, you are overweight or obese.

So let's have a 'keeping it real' moment. YOU are the thick chick. Your senior year of high school people start to notice your figure. Then, you go to off to college or to the military. Can't tell you nothing. You are "sho'nuff" fine. All through your late twenties, you don't have to work at all to show why you're a brick house, baby! By the time you hit your thirties, you are still eating the same as you did in your late teens to early twenties. You start to notice your clothes are fitting a tad bit tighter. No worries, you just go up a size. By the time you hit your forties, life has happened. For some, you have a husband (or an ex-husband), children and a career you may or may not be satisfied with after several years on the job. Maybe you've even lost a loved one. All of this can be overwhelming. At this point, you are no longer a thick chick. That time has come and gone. Now the weight gain has started to affect your health.

So back to the "keeping it real" moment. You, my friend CANNOT continue down this path. This is a path of neglect and unhealthy choices. You're too important. How many dress sizes must you go up over a ten-year period? Decide right now to commit to your well -being. I am not asking you to become the skinny chick, but I am asking you to be the woman who deserves to live an excellent healthy existence.

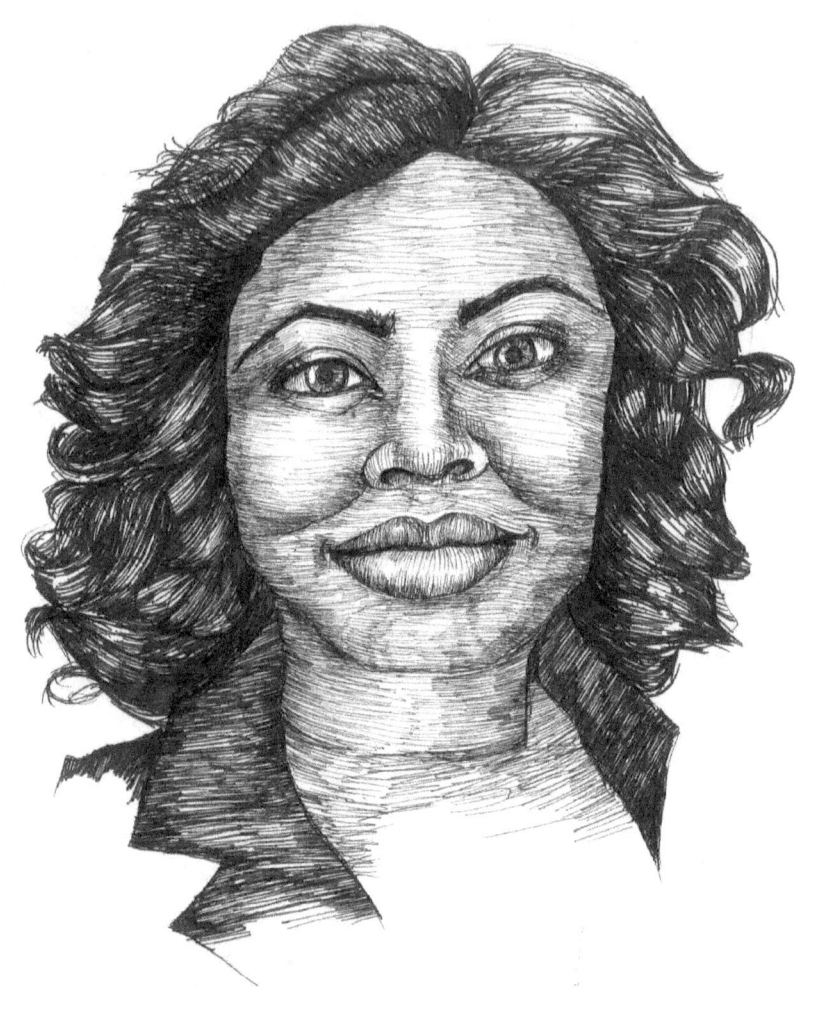

Chapter 7

What's this health thing worth to you?

Everything has a cost. Nothing is free. Even when people say they will give you a free gift just for listening to a presentation, you know you're not going to buy it, but it will cost you your time. So again, nothing is free in this life. Everything has a price. So, I ask you what is your health worth to you?

For example, how much is a good sports bra worth to you? I have heard women say they don't want to work out because their breasts are large and it's just not comfortable for them. Their breast jiggle or bounce up and down when they try to work out. I totally get that. But what I would strongly suggest is investing in a very good sports bra. A good sports bra is not going to be found at your local big box retailer. You need to go somewhere where you can be measured. Get a bra that compresses and that also will encapsulate each breast. This will create stability and deliver support. A good sports bra can do wonders for your bouncy breasts while you work out. Of course, it will also benefit your total body. You may need to speak to your doctor as well. If your breasts are hurting your back and your bra straps are leaving indentations, you may very well be medically qualified for breast reduction surgery.

What is spending a little time outside worth to you? I hate to go here, but I must. Unfortunately, as a physical education teacher who has worked with thousands of students over several years, I have heard way too many students say "Mrs. K.C. I don't want to go outside. I am going to get black." Or, "I don't want to get too dark, do we have to go outside today?" My next question to my students is always, what wrong with being Black? They basically give something of the same routine answer. "It's nothing wrong, but I don't want to get too dark."

Or, occasionally I will hear students say their mom does not want them to stay outside to long because "she wants me to stay my same complexion." This use to be a 'Wow' moment for me, because it was hard to believe people still thought like this, especially young people. Even though they may not realize it, subconsciously an adult in their life has taught them two very sad and perhaps disastrous lessons. One, if your skin color is dark, you are not beautiful or attractive. And two, any outdoor activity--including much needed exercise--is a no go. Yes, it's true slavery has produced generations of negative psychological effects that are still perpetuated today.

I realize there are some people who just can't take the heat, especially as we get older. For those women, it's important to work out in the early morning or late evening, when the sun is not at its peak. And don't forget sunscreen. Yes, Black folks need sunscreen! Exercising will not always take place in a nice air conditioned gym or equipment filled home. It's good to go outside and walk, run, play, exercise and get some fresh air. Please, let's not just say no to exercising outside simply because of this notion that the sun will make me dark and ugly. This is rooted in self -hate. Also, for goodness sakes, please stop infiltrating our children's mind with such foolishness.

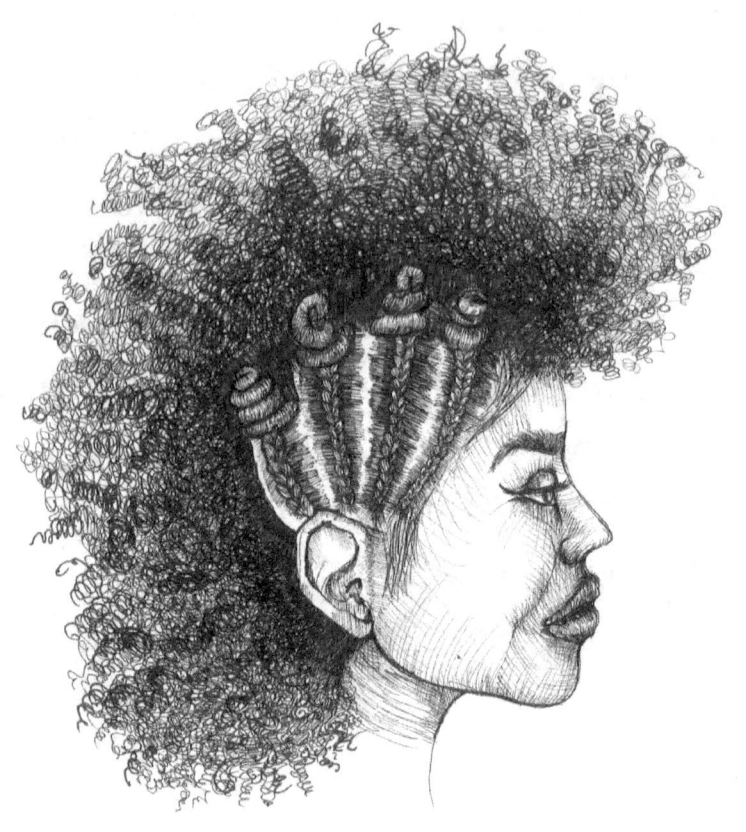

Chapter 8

We all have to leave here but…

Back in 2010, talk show host Oprah Winfrey hosted an episode of her show that detailed the effects obesity can have on individuals even after death. The show discussed how caskets are increasing in size to accommodate the growing number of obese remains that funeral homes are now preparing. So even in death, obesity can cost you and your loved ones financially.

It's tough to bury a loved one. It's emotional, heartbreaking and the grief can be overwhelming. If it's a really close loved one, it can feel like a piece of you is gone forever. We bury them, but we live with the wonderful memories. Clearly, since you are reading this book you are not buried. Instead, you're allowing a seed to be planted. Pastor Dale Bronner said that being planted and buried are both in the same place, underneath the ground. However, if you are planted, there is opportunity for growth. If you are buried, it's over for you and your growth here on Earth is done.

Plants and vegetables don't just pop out of the ground when they are planted. It's a slow process. But they do grow. Your growth will be a process as well. But this growth, if you allow it, will have wonderful benefits. Taking control of your health, your body, your mind, the foods you put in your body and getting good exercise will provide proactive and preventive benefits that will change your life.

For it is true, we are born to die. None of us will live forever. But what is so critical is what we do for ourselves and our loved ones while we are here on Earth. Ask yourself this question, 'What kind of habits I am teaching my children?' Are you preparing them to be able to eat to live and not live to eat? Believe it or not, what you teach your children about food, (e.g., how to prepare healthy meals, appropriate portion sizes, and what's nurturing to their bodies) is a part of the legacy you leave for your offspring--as well as future generations.

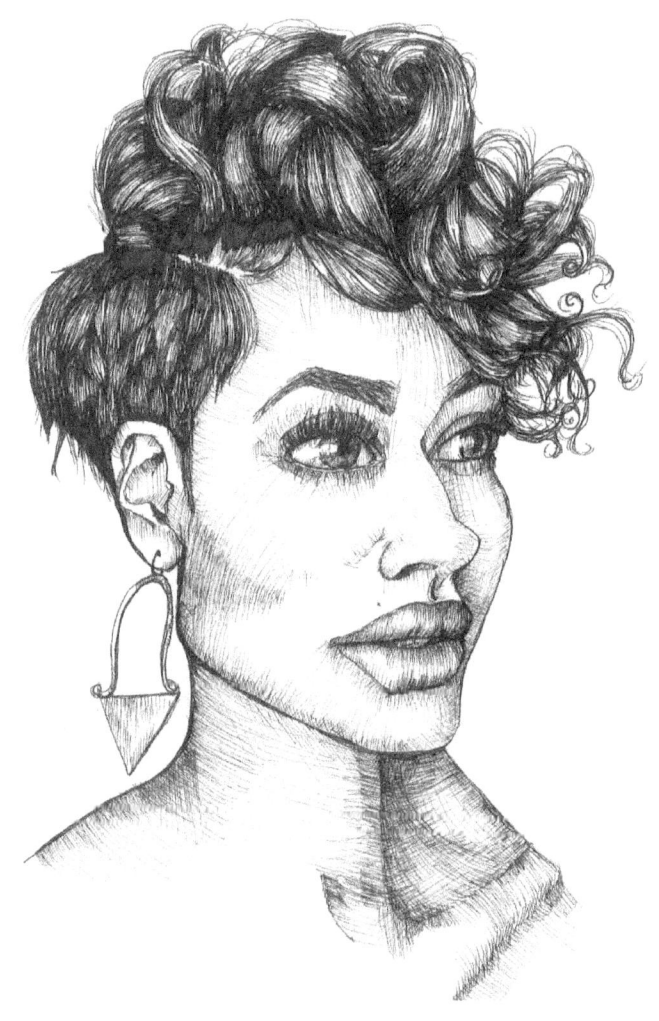

Chapter 9

Execution

The benefits of exercise and a healthy diet have been well documented. This guidebook is designed to help you understand how critical it is to reduce the number of overweight and obese woman and help reduce the risk of preventable illnesses. However; there are also many other benefits. According to the Centers for Disease Control, they include helping maintain healthy bones, muscles and joints, reducing symptoms of anxiety and depression, reduction in some types of cancers and preventing premature death.

At the beginning of the book, I touched on the concept of excuses verses execution. Now, let's elaborate. There will be no more excuses for you. It's time to execute a growth plan that will have a lasting impact on you and those around you. Once others around you see you working toward a change, they will want to be a part of the change that is taking place in you.

One of the most beautiful things I see when I go back home to Atlanta are these amazing group of women playing kickball in leagues all around the city and surrounding suburbs. They are gettin' it! I see them practicing on Sunday after church. I see them playing in their leagues and they are having fun. These women are all shapes and sizes. Some are athletic, some are not; it does not matter. No excuses, just execution of the willingness to play and enjoy the camaraderie of other sister friends.

Kickball may not be your thing, but how about walking? Start off by walking around the block. It is a simple first step. Next, when you go to the grocery store or your nearest big box retailer don't drive around looking for the closest parking space. Park as far back in the parking lot as you can and walk in. If you have stairs at work, walk or jog those. Next, go into your local mall or outside the mall. Many people forget about the mall. But this a great place- especially in the early morning because there is usually mall security driving around the parking lot to ensure all is well. Walking inside the mall can be beneficial as well, particularly during the peak of summer and winter months when the temperatures are extremely hot or extremely cold. Walking inside the mall can offer a safe, air conditioned or warm, cozy environment.

Walking at a local park is always an option. However, make sure the park is full of other walkers or take a partner with you. It is never a good idea to walk alone. Speaking of walking with a partner, which is a great idea, why not get the whole family involved? Take the kids, husband, grandma, friend, whoever is nearby and do it together. Walking with your significant other or children is also a time to bond. Great conversations can take place during this time. If your child or children are toddlers, put them in a stroller and get to moving. Remember it's about executing a plan and leaving the excuses behind.

Another place you may consider for exercise is the local middle or junior high and high school. Every community is different, but many times these schools have a track and field that is not being utilized before or after a certain time of day. For example, in the early morning before school starts, you may be able to get some laps in or in the evening after you get off work. After football, soccer, and track practice have ended, the facilities may be open to the public. If these options are available, start walking around the track. On a regulation size track, four times around is a mile. Ideas of how to execute a plan are in full effect.

Church is where we go to get our praise on and to renew and charge up for the upcoming week. For some time now, many churches have become the place where not just the spirit is being fed and taken care of, but is also the place where the physical body can go and get exercise. The church has been the corner stone of the African American community, dating all the way back to slavery through the Civil Rights Movement. The church's role has always been substantial and extremely significant for African Americans. Some may argue that the church's role has diminished. I whole heartily disagree. I am increasingly seeing African American churches stepping up and taking a lead in trying to get their members active and healthy.

Family Life Centers are being built and not only church members are encouraged to attend but also those from the surrounding community are invited to join and be a part of this health and wellness movement. Many of these Family Life Centers offer work out classes such as Zumba, yoga, step aerobics and boot camps. Some have swimming pools and several offer exercise equipment rooms where you can find tread mills, step up machines and other aerobics equipment. Some offer weight rooms as well. Many churches that do not have workout facilities are still starting to offer classes for their members. It's great to see these churches actively involved in promoting good health and wellness for their congregation and other members of the community.

If you are still not feeling any of these options, then try your local recreation (rec) department. The rec department in many counties and districts are taking a lead in their communities. Many offer classes that are reasonably priced. Go ahead, call them up and see what programs they have to offer.

Local community gyms are great. Many times, staff members there get to know the clientele on a personal level and can make a tremendous difference in their lives. Often times, it is smaller and the trainers and workers take the time to provide the best service to the customer. You're not just a number coming to workout, you're a person who is working to get real results. Trainers at the smaller health gyms usually understand this and make every effort to help you reach your goals.

At larger franchise health clubs with more name recognition, you get a lot. More equipment, bigger facility, more class offerings. These larger workout places can be a social meat market as well, which can be a distraction, deterrent or even a motivation. Your comfort level will determine what works best for you. These facilities will cost more, but provide quite a bit and they stay open later than the rec centers and many local gyms. Some of these fitness health clubs are open 24 hours a day, seven days a week.

High end health clubs are out of this world. They cost, but boy are they nice. Many have spas, nutrition services with gourmet meals, as well as Swedish, deep tissue and many other types of massages. They offer state of the art playrooms for children. The trainers there will cost more, but you're not only paying for what the trainers are able to offer or teach. You're paying for the ambiance, that comes with being in a high-end health, wellness and fitness club.

If you are looking for something that is family oriented and will suit the needs of all family members, the local YMCA is the place for you. I love the Y. It's like a one stop shop. They have activities for the kids while you work out. You can sign the kids up for different sports and at some locations they offer martial arts. While the kids practice the sport of their choice, you can exercise. Some offer nutrition classes that focus on diabetes prevention and many other wonderful options for the entire family. I have also found that most YMCA's also make sure they take care of their senior citizen population. They have special events and programs that are specifically designed for seniors. They love it! The Y has something for everybody—including you.

If you need a little extra help, reputable medical weight loss and wellness centers are also a viable option. These places offer a board-certified physician to hold your hand and walk you through the steps you need to reach a healthy weight and live a healthy lifestyle.

Some neighborhoods or apartment complexes also offer workout rooms. They may or may not compare to the previously mentioned options, but at least it's a start. Why not give it a try if it's available to you?

Make a decision to start somewhere. Even if that somewhere is just walking to the mailbox, then to the corner and back. Plant a garden and work in your garden. It may not seem like it, but gardening is a great physical activity. There are many ways to get your exercise.

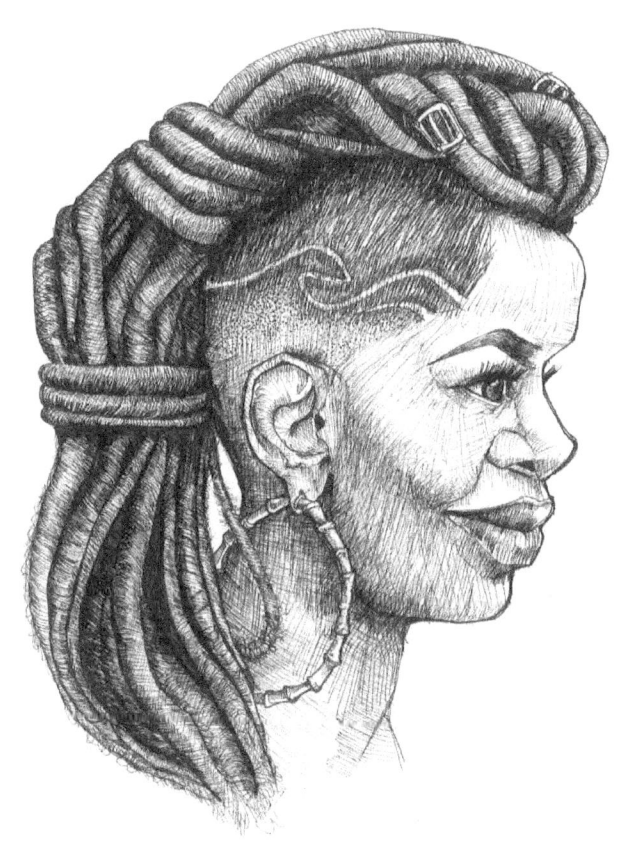

Chapter 10

What my mommy taught me.

The following texts were written by my children. I asked them to write something they felt reflected what they have been taught by elders in the family, myself and their wonderful father—who has been my fitness partner for nearly twenty years. There was no prompting or prodding to get them to say anything except their true thoughts.

Nine year old daughter, Nia

Hi. I am the author's daughter. My mommy has been a PE teacher for a lot of years. She taught me to always stay active and eat my veggies.
My mommy also taught me to stay healthy by not watching TV all the time and going outside and playing soccer or racing and any other sport you love. Sometimes I don't want to do it, but once we start playing, it's fine.

Twelve year old son, Rod

Hello, I am the author's son. When it comes to eating, my mom says it is okay to have a treat every once in a while, but you shouldn't just eat treats and go out and eat all the time. You have to balance your diet out and eat vegetables and fruits and maybe eat a salad when you go out. My mom cooks healthy dishes most of the time, but on some days she will cook hamburgers and French fries. What she does is balance out our diet so we eat healthy most of the time and "rewards" us like every two weeks. Also, she takes us to work out like 3 or 4 days of the week. Most of the time we go running but sometimes we will go as a family to the YMCA and we will go in a room and do exercises like push-ups or sit ups. She is balancing out our diet and to add on to that our workouts.

Now that you've heard from my children, I encourage you to examine what you are teaching your children. By getting up and out and participating in physical activity, you send a powerful message to your children—one that you are not only telling, but also practicing. Also, examine how you handle the food you eat. For example, when you sit down to eat do you automatically pour salt on your food without even tasting it to see if it needs of any salt? This is a habit that you should break. Taste the food first, it could be seasoned just right. No need to add salt where it may not be needed.

Okay my sister…Just one more thought. Like the ancestors who came before you, you were built for greatness! There are some things in life you may not be able to prevent. However, when it comes to preventable illnesses, you must take the lead in your health. Do NOT allow preventable illnesses to hamper you from being and doing great things. I hope this guide will help you jump-start the journey that leads to the best and most wonderful version of YOU.

No judgement here, my only goal is to give you practical strategies for losing weight, improving your health and changing your life. On this journey, you must be honest with yourself. You must be ready to change your behavior. I want you to love the woman you discover at the end of this journey--and love her enough to care for her as well as you care for everyone else in your life.

So, come on, beautiful--let's move! No more excuses! It's time to execute your new plan to make good health and great physical fitness your top priorities!

Thank You

"If you have never experienced any troubles in your life, keep living." I've heard that expression countless times over the years and eventually realized life's troubles almost always become growth experiences. Sometimes these experiences will knock the very breath out of you--leaving you dazed, confused, lost and begging God to do something to make the pain go away. Yet, somehow, some way...you manage to get back up, start over or simply create a new normal.

I have had to create a new normal since my mother, Geraldine Calhoun Kerr, transitioned to her heavenly home in 2016. Fortunately, I had a lot of help picking up the pieces and getting to the point to where I could turn a test into a testimony. To that end, I must thank those who have helped me along in this journey of life.

The Kerrs, the Calhouns, and the Jackson families make up the village that raised me, and in later years, the Conleys helped enrich that village. I am grateful and thankful for each and every member of my family. From the time that I was in my mother's womb and after I carried two in my own womb, you all have loved, supported and encouraged me every step of the way.

My beloved sorors of Delta Sigma Theta have laughed with me, cried with me and travelled across the Earth with me. I love you all dearly--especially the sorors of my beloved Eta Chapter. To my Fort Valley State University family, thank you for helping to mold me into the woman and fitness expert I am today. The seeds of friendship planted on that campus in Fort Valley, Georgia have blossomed into priceless relationships that have carried me through the years. Thank you, Dr. Skip Valois, by way of Dr. William Zimmerli and the University of South Carolina Arnold School of Public Health, for helping me discover the tools I would need to be an effective public health educator. Special thanks to Portia Bruner for challenging and questioning me while we edited this manuscript over laughs and tears at my parents' dining room table.

To Dr. Krystal L. Conner, Dr. Fredly Bataille and Chiquitta Gosha, thank you for your help and insight and the funny conversions we shared as I progressed in writing this book. Thank you, Meme Norris and Latonya Tripp -Dinkins for your support and enduring love and friendship. Thank you, Ebony Johnson, for your lifelong friendship. You introduced me to Marcus Howell and for that, I am forever grateful. Thank you,

Marcus, for showing me how to navigate the business of book publishing. To my church family First Baptist on Gresham Road in Atlanta, Georgia, thank you for your prayers and support.

To my little brother, Dr. Jelani C. Kerr, I love you and thank you for your continued support. You are a brilliant man and I am fortunate to have your insight and sense of pragmatism in my life.

To my little sister, Dr. Shantia K. Sims, you mean everything to me. There are no words. I'm truly thankful God saw fit to make you my sister, my friend, and my biggest cheerleader. Even when I would present you with the most outlandish ideas, you always assure me that I can and WILL do it. Love you to life, forever!

Next to Jesus, I don't believe a better man has walked the Earth than my daddy. Paul Kerr is the best father a girl could ever have. I love you, daddy. Thank you for showing me a how man is supposed to treat his wife and the mother of his children. Thank you being a model of Agape love and showing me how to be respectful-- even when I am struggling to do so.

To my son, Roderick Conley, (a.k.a. Great) and my daughter Nia (a.k.a Nia-Bell), thank you for being a constant source of unfiltered joy, true love and sheer amazement. Mommy loves you. God has awesome plans for your life. Remember to always remain grateful and humble.

Last, but certainly not least, I must cast a million thank you's to my wonderful husband Roderick Conley (Big Rod). He is my friend, my work out partner, my head coach (or assistant coach depending on my mood before the game) and my rock! Rod, you are absolutely the real deal--truly one of

Decatur's Greatest! I love you more than
I did on the first day of our marriage.
Through all the tough times and the
phenomenal times, I could always count
on you to have my back. I look forward
to many more wonderful years together.
I thank the Most High for you. Love you
Rod…today and for the rest of our lives!

And finally, to my wonderful
mother, Geraldine Calhoun Kerr. I truly
thank God for your life—a life well
lived. You taught me to love education,
not to quit and how a true champion
must fight and never give up. A winner
is what I call you. You battled cancer
three times and came out on top. You are
still winning as you now have your
heavenly crown with our Lord and
Savior. Thank you Ma, for your
continued support. Even though we did
not always see eye to eye you never gave
up on me. I also call you tough. You
would say what you meant and meant

what you said. Everybody knew
Geraldine didn't play. Love ya, Ma!

Afterword

By Tissilli Rogers
Owner of TissFit, Atlanta, Georgia
Certified Personal Trainer

In my ten plus years as a personal trainer I have helped many clients achieve their personal fitness goals. Those that made a heartfelt decision to put the time and work in achieved impressive results. Those that gave more excuses than effort, not so much. As a fitness expert, I know firsthand deciding to make permanent habit and lifestyle changes can have a profound impact upon a person. Come On Beautiful, Move! should be used as a tool to motivate change in a mindset. Transforming your mind will not only help to mold you into what you desire but will also help to increase your intrinsic value.

So often we search, but are not entirely sure where to find the tools that will help us live a healthy lifestyle. If we don't know where to find answers, we start to look extrinsically. Hard earned money will be spent on waist shapers, pantyhose that give the illusion of a healthy body, and other temporary fixes. The time for microwave results are over. Your children and other love ones model the behaviors they see. Why not show them something that is real and long lasting and will be a blessing to the next generation?

Working to achieve optimal health from the outside in will not have lasting results. It's fleeting and will leave you in a cycle that is extremely difficult to overcome. But you can overcome. Education is the key, along with desire, discipline, and a strong will to do better. Come On Beautiful, Move! is the educational piece that will point you in the right direction. It is enlightening and an agent of change that will help you to create new habits and a better you.

Stay inspired as you go on this journey to attain your best you. Others see you and are depending upon you. Don't get caught up in what others are doing on social media. Everything or everybody is not as it appears. If you need inspiration, reread this book and be guided by the principles that have been offered. Remember, you can achieve lasting, excellent health.

Work Cited

"CFR-Code of Federal Regulation Title 21." Accessdata.fda.gov. N.p., 01 Apr. 2016. Web. 06 Apr.2017.

Gathers, Raechele; Mahan, Meredith. African American Women, Hair Care, and Health Barriers. The Journal of Clinical and Aesthetic Dermatology. 2014 September; Volume 7 (NO. 9): 26-29

Hall, Rebecca MD; Francis, Shani, MD, MBA; Whitt-Glover, Melicia, Ph.D; Loftin-Bell, Kismet, MS; Swett, Katrina, MS; McMichael, J. Amy, MD. Hair Care Practices as a Barrier to Physical Activity in African American Women. JAMA Dermatol. 2013; VOL 149 (NO.3): 310-314

Obesity and African Americans. (2016, June 24). Retrieved June 27, 2016, from https://minorityhealth.hhs.gov/omh/browse.aspx?lvl=4&lvlid=25

Pallarito, Karen. (2011, April 11)."Weaves, Braids May Speed Hair Loss in Black Women - CNN.com." Retrieved from http://www.cnn.com/2011/HEALTH/04/11/br aids.weaves.hair.loss/index.html CNN.com - N.p., n.d. Web. 19 Oct. 2016.

Pekmezi, Dori; Marcus,Bes;, Menesses; Karen; Baskin L. Monica; Ard, D. Jamy; Martin Y. Michelle; Adams, Natasia; Robinson, Cody; Demark-Wahnefried. Developing an intervention to address physical activity barriers for African-American women in the deep south (USA). Womens Health (Long Engl). 2013 May; ((3): 301-12.(PubMed: 23638785)

www.ingramcontent.com/pod-product-compliance
Lightning Source LLC
Chambersburg PA
CBHW071217280526
45787CB00002B/710